I0441804

Talking with Your Physician by Lawrence W. Gold, M.D. Originally published April 2013 as I Love My Doctor, but…

A Grass Valley Publishing Production
Cartoons by Theresa Mccracken (mchumor@pioneer.net)

First edition February 2016
Printed in the United States of America

# Dedication

**To my wife, Dorlis**

**When I suggested my first non-fiction book, she was supportive, as usual, and said, "Go for it."**

## Acknowledgments

Dawné Dominique, a gifted artist and cover designer for help with the cover.

Donna Meares, editing.

Tony Lesce and Margaret Gold for their reviews and suggestions.

Theresa Mccracken, a gifted cartoonist.

**Works By Lawrence W. Gold, M.D.**

**Fiction—Brier Hospital Series:**

First, Do No Harm

No Cure for Murder

The Sixth Sense

Tortured Memory

The Plague Within

Trapped

Hybrid

Never Too Late

State of Mind

The Doctors' Lounge

Out of Darkness

**Other Novels:**

For the Love of God

Rage

Deadly Passage

A Simple Cure

**Non-Fiction:**

Talking with your Physician (Surviving Obamacare)

All available in print, Kindle, and most as audiobooks.

# Author's Note

If you're among the millions of patients who have a good relationship with your physician, this book may not be for you. In that case, you have my congratulations. Cherish and protect that association for the medicine of the future may make that relationship increasingly problematic.

While I hope readers will enjoy this small book, it has serious intent as well. It deals with a pressing issue of our time, the provision of healthcare. The full implementation of the Affordable Care Act (ACA or Obamacare), makes this information even more important. The ACA is a compromise, perhaps the only one feasible for our times, but it's a troublesome one at that. I have hope that it will work out its bugs. As a more than satisfied Medicare recipient, I hope, some day, to see Medicare for all or its equivalent.

We're watching a war between two different approaches for paying for healthcare: government based and market based systems. Unfortunately, arguments about paying for healthcare have fallen smack into the political arena where ideology and power are more important than providing and improving care.

If we want to save money and provide good medical care, we should focus on the patient and his/her physician. Within that relationship is the pathway to providing healthcare that doctors and patients want, and society can afford.

This book may be more useful today than it was the first time I thought about writing it. I'd been thinking about how patients and their physicians got along, what's wrong with it, and how to make it better.

—

I've left the major healthcare issues for other's books (take your choice from the thousands). Providers, insurers, healthcare administrators, and politicians of every stripe have their own ideas about how to fix our healthcare system, but for the most part, they focus on how to pay for it.

I won't apologize for some repetitive material in this book because my aim is twofold: to educate and to persuade. The latter suggests coming at issues in different ways until I convince the reader to consider their value.

# OBAMACARE

One wonders why the Affordable Care Act (Obamacare) that provides healthcare
to millions lacking coverage, and eliminates major health insurance
deficiencies, such as denying coverage for preexisting conditions, has been
characterized as the most polarizing political legislation in decades. As
Groucho Marx said, "Politics is the art of looking for trouble, finding it
everywhere, diagnosing it incorrectly, and employing the wrong remedies."

Regardless of political persuasion, providing medical care to all who need it, via
the Affordable Care Act or any other system, will result in exactly the same
set of problems:

- Many more people will require care:
- The ACA enrolled over eight million of which, over seven million are still
  subscribers.
- More patients can overwhelm our already overburdened providers:
- Over 80 percent of physicians are overextended or working at full capacity.
- More patient care in the face of uncontrolled healthcare inflation can stress or
  bankrupt the system or the individual: effective cost containment, an intrinsic
  part of the system, has yet to come to full fruition.
- More patient care may not mean better care, in fact, it may make outcomes
  worse (see below).
- Medical care is in transition to Accountable Care, a system to designed to
  reduce hospital admissions, specialty care, readmissions, and to encourage
  prevention. While these goals are laudable, elements may be destructive to
  the practice of medicine itself. Providers not meeting goals are guilty until
  they prove themselves innocent, choice suffers, and limiting referrals has the
  potential to harm patients.

The overriding message is: If you have a physician, make your relationship work for the both of you—you're in this together. If you don't have a physician, get one as soon as possible, but remember, you may be in trouble as even mediocre ones may be hard to find (See conclusions).

## Personal Note

I've been a physician in the U.S. Army in Vietnam, private office and hospital-based practices, and have served as chief of a large department of internal medicine and family practice.

While from time to time, the media targets physicians for greed, mistakes, and attitude, still medicine scores high in surveys of the most respected professions, deservedly so, in my opinion. Largely, the physicians I've known rank high in those character traits people cherish the most: intelligence, dedication, honesty, and integrity.

# Quotations

- If you have more surgeons, you'll get more surgery. If you have more internists, you'll get more lab tests. ( John Wennberg )

- We shall have to learn to refrain from doing things merely because we know how to do them.  ( Theodore Fox )

- Be careful about reading health books. You may die of a misprint. ( or updated: may die of an Internet glitch)  ( Mark Twain )

- I recently became a Christian Scientist. It was the only health plan I could afford.

- ( Betsy Salkind )

- According to a new report, more than 700 fake Obamacare websites have been created. Security experts say it's simple to identify the phony sites because they are easy to log on to.

- (Jay Leno)

- If you wouldn't want it done to you, don't do it to your patient.

- ( Lawrence W. Gold, M.D. )

- The doctor is the only man who can suffer from good health.

- (anon)

# TABLE OF CONTENTS

- FORWARD
- INTRODUCTION
- THE PROBLEMS
- I HATE DOCTORS NARRATIVES
- PATIENT AND PHYSICIAN COMMUNICATION
- QUESTIONS FOR PHYSICIANS AND PATIENTS
- ESSENTIAL QUESTIONS FOR PATIENTS
- MEDICAL MALPRACTICE
- MATCHING PATIENT AND PHYSICIAN
- BE CAREFUL WHAT YOU WISH FOR
- THE "MORE IS ALWAYS BETTER" PHILOSOPHY
- MEDICAL PROBLEMS THAT PHYSICIAN DISLIKE
- FINDING A PHYSICIAN
- MEDICAL MYTHS
- THE PROBLEMS WITH MEDICAL ADVICE
- INTRODUCTION TO MEDICAL TERMINOLOGY
- COMPUTERS AND THE DOCTOR-PATIENT RELATIONSHIP
- FINDING ANSWERS ONLINE
- CONCLUSIONS
- SAVING THE RELATIONSHIP WITH YOUR PHYSICIAN
- WHEN SHOULD YOU FIRE YOUR DOCTOR
- MAKING THE RIGHT DECISIONS ABOUT EMERGENCY CARE
- GLOSSARY OF MEDICAL TERMINOLOGY
- GLOSSARY OF MEDICAL SPECIALISTS

# FOREWARD

More than fifty years ago, in April of 1965, Dr. Morton Bogdonoff, the
Chief Editor of JAMA, the Journal of the American Medical
Association, wrote this abstract:

During the past several years, one of the criticisms leveled at the
practice of medicine in modern day America has been the
supposed loss of the "old personal touch" from the doctor-
patient relationship. These criticisms have been noted in
both professional and lay publications, and have indicated
that the blame is often leveled specifically at the increase in
subspecialization, as well as at the use of complicated and
intricate diagnostic procedures that entail much technical
time, leaving little for physician-patient interactions. Many
of these communications have a tone of longing for the
"good old days" and the physician of "horse and buggy"
renown. Though the physician and patient may well have
known each other much more intimately in years past, the
"good old days" were perhaps not so "good," and one would
hardly wish to return to a less effective type of medical
practice.

Recently, I have spent time making rounds at a university hospital.
While hospitals have streamlined their medical wards with
computer systems that increase accuracy, deliver information
rapidly, and keep track of diagnostic information, both current
and past, my overall impression was not too dissimilar from
previous experience. The intensive care unit had, in my day,
acute care nurses at the bedside of the sickest patients. Today,

however, nurses, physicians, and auxiliary medical personnel spend an inordinate amount of time before the computer, rather than at the bedside. This observation does not impugn the care they provide; it suggests that the current state of the art for the application of the computer to medical care has a way to go.

# INTRODUCTION

If you trust Google more than your doctor, maybe it's time to switch doctors. (Jadelr and Cristina Cordova)

As if we don't have enough trouble in American life, economics, changing attitudes, and pressures suggest that it's time for us to deal with problems between patients and their doctors. It's easy to find guilt; just look at greedy doctors, ignorant and demanding patients, and the dysfunctional healthcare system. Oscar Wilde said it best: "It's not whether you win or lose, it's how you place the blame."

In addition, we have the Internet, a savior and a Pandora's Box (see computers in medicine).

The problems cited in this book are more than inconvenient or undesirable; they have a direct impact on both physicians and their patients. Specifically, these conflicts affect patients' lives, health, and—hold your hats— the cost of providing medical care.

*Relationship* (how I'm getting to hate that word) has become an overworked catchphrase. A Google keyword search on "relationship" produces over eleven million hits per month. Our major relationships, interpersonal, clergy, and with our physicians, have taken a hit, especially as we've seen patient-doctor relationships complaints increasing each year.

To paraphrase Shakespeare, the fault lies not only in our HMOs, PPOs, or in the Affordable Care Act, but in ourselves. These systems don't make things any easier for physicians and their patients, but the need for medical care isn't going away, and most physicians still enjoy

—

treating their patients. Improving medical care may be beyond the capability of our dysfunctional government and insurance industry, so, the trick, for the moment at least, may be to make do, or at least, not make things worse.

Often, it feels as if the world is conspiring against patients and physicians as politicians, insurance companies, and lawmakers complicate, confound, and challenge the relationship we'd all like to have with our physicians. I'm not talking about nostalgia for good times past where, for instance, the TV program *Medic* (1954-1956) opened with the announcer's dedication to physicians as, guardians of birth, healers of the sick, comforters of the aged..."

The entertainment industry of the sixties and seventies produced the doctors we still yearn for today. The world (especially women) loved Dr. Kildare, Ben Casey, and Marcus Welby, but objective analysis of their behaviors would find them falling short in today's world, especially in their patronizing attitudes toward women. A 1971 Episode of Marcus Welby was entitled, "A Woman's Place..."

If you've lived long enough, you can remember the kindly, caring, self-sacrificing, humanistic, physicians who were unfailingly compassionate. How many physicians today live up to that ideal or even want to?

In May of 2007, Donna Karen wrote in the *Huffington Post*: Where is Marcus Welby, MD?

Nostalgia is great, but it won't get us the care we deserve, and it won't satisfy physicians who, even today, despite barriers, still thrive on helping their patients.

# THE PROBLEMS

- Unrealistic expectations on all sides.

- The logistics of being a patient or a doctor.

- Malpractice litigation.

- Demands of healthcare insurers.

- Destructive attitudes:
Physician towards patient.
Patient towards physician.

- The almighty dollar (too much or too little).

- The profit motive in healthcare.

"THIS WILL ONLY HURT FOR A MOMENT."

## I HATE DOCTORS NARRATIVES
(How can you fix a problem that you don't understand?)

**My doctor is nice; every time I see him, I'm ashamed of what I think of doctors in general. (Mignon McLaughlin)**

I shouldn't have been surprised, but I was. Below are representative results of an Internet search on the phrase, "I hate doctors."

While I, and most physicians would find these examples unrepresentative and dismiss them, these comments, while extreme, intemperate, inaccurate, or just plain nuts, suggest that we would be smart to focus on their factual and emotional content, and ask, as they do in women's magazines, "Can this relationship be saved?"

If you're a physician, your reaction to these narratives will be similar to mine, but these opinions exist, and to some, they reflect a subset of reality.

These narratives are selected from actual comments on the Internet. I've partially edited, and paraphrased them to protect the innocent/guilty:

## NARRATIVE I

I hate doctors because they do not care about what happens to their patients, they do not listen to their patients, they are rude, they pretend they are better than their patients, and they do not care about their patients' concerns. It is difficult to feel any kind of respect for someone like that.

It's rare to find doctors who actually care and don't talk down to their patients and can help patients in a meaningful way. I have never met a doctor who took feedback as an indication of how they were doing with their patients. Most interpret constructive criticism as a complaint or a threat. That puts them on the defensive and deprives them of a reality check on how they're practicing. It should be a wakeup call that has the potential to make them more humane since they are, in essence, heartless, soulless, cold, calculating creatures.

## NARATIVE II

I can't express how much I hate doctors. The only time I will see one is when I am absolutely forced to, and only when someone else will pay the bill.

Every illness I have ever suffered cost me thousands of dollars in tests and doctor visits. First, they always keep me waiting, and afterward, they bounced me from one specialist to another at the cost of thousands more. I think they conspire with each other. Besides not listening, they don't believe what I say. Can you imagine how that feels? In the end, it's always a disease that any first year medical student could have diagnosed in thirty seconds.

—

# Comment

Before we reject these critical observations as out-to-lunch, we should
review objective studies of patient satisfaction where we will find,
without the vitriol, some interesting correlations. Overall, complaints
against physicians are up by 23% plus, mostly against general
practitioners and psychiatrists.

Note that while complaints (gripes may be a better word) are more
common against family practitioners and psychiatrists, lawsuits are
more common against neurosurgeons, cardio-thoracic surgeons,
general surgeons, family practitioners, and pediatricians (in that
order). While it's clear that surgeons deal with higher-risk patients
and worse outcomes, other factors may come into play, such as more
dramatic bad outcomes, easier prosecution, deeper pockets, and the
tendency of malpractice insurance companies to settle claims.

In rough order of frequency, these are the complaints:

- Waiting too long to get an appointment for an office visit.
- Too much time sitting in the waiting room.
- Physicians spent too little time with patients and didn't explain enough.
- Didn't call with test results or return phone calls,
- Lacked compassion.
- Showed disrespectful and rude behavior.
- Didn't listen to their patients, especially regarding what they've learned from reading, talking to others, or from the Internet.
- Don't believe their patients, or worse, think they're nuts.
- Take your choice: The physician refers too often or too rarely.
- Doctors disdain non-traditional medicine. They think they know everything.

# PATIENT AND PHYSICIAN COMMUNICATIONS
# THE CORNERSTONE OF MEDICINE

**There is only one cardinal rule: One must always listen to the patient.**
**Oliver Sacks**

An old joke about communications and medical language helps make the
point:

"Doc," says Steve, "I want to be castrated."

"What on earth for?"

"It's something I've been thinking about for a long time. If you don't do it,
I'll just go to another doctor."

"OK, but it's against my better judgment."

Steve has his operation. The next day he walks down the hospital corridor
very slowly, legs apart.

Heading toward him is another patient walking exactly the same way.

"Hi there," says Steve, "It looks as if you've just had the same operation as
me."

"Yeah," says the patient, "I finally decided I'd like to be circumcised."

Steve's eyes widen in horror, "Oh no! That's the word!"

## Doctors and Patients Don't Know How to Talk with Each Other

Even before we had the data, both physicians and their patients knew intuitively that communication between them was important. Clinicians, epidemiologists, university medical programs, and patient advocates filled the medical and general literature with studies describing the relationship, its deficiencies and recommendations for improvement.

Today, we know without question that better communication leads to more physician and patient satisfaction and improved outcomes. These outcomes, for example, include better control of high blood pressure, improved glucose control in diabetics, and less frequent episodes of asthma and congestive heart failure. A word before we get into communications: the medical literature contains many references to patient compliance or non-compliance, that is, how well patients follow their doctor's instructions.

Compliance, like the word tolerance, carries unintended meanings. When I hear of religious tolerance, for instance, it registers in my head as "put up with," and when physicians talk about compliance, it suggests a subservient relationship between the patient and the physician. Synonyms aren't much better: accede, acquiesce, cave in, come around, consent to, and my all time favorite, cry uncle. Well-meaning healthcare advocates have even suggested the word concordance, but to my ears that sounds like an edict from the pope.

Let's give "adhere to" a shot. Substitute "comply," if you must.

"I DON'T KNOW WHAT YOUR PROBLEM IS.
MY PATIENTS ALWAYS FOLLOW MY ORDERS."

## Good communications means:

- Office visits are less threatening and more pleasurable for patient and physician.
- Diagnosis improves.
- Treatment is appropriate to the patient's condition.
- Adherence to recommendations for treatment and/or medications improves.
- Outcomes improve.
- Malpractice claims lessen.
- Physicians practice less defensively.
- Physician and patient frustration in the face of difficult medical problems are lessened.

While it's clear that these are qualitative improvements for docs and their patients, the economic impact is equally clear. For instance, sources estimate that non-adherence to physician recommendations costs somewhere between $100 billion and $289 billion dollars each year and results in 10 percent of hospital admissions. (The Atlantic Sept. 11, 2012)

Think of the human cost as well

## Whose Life is it, Anyway?

Speaking up to your physician and/or following his/her recommendations are the most important things that patients can do for their health and well being. Yet, getting some patients to speak up and comply is difficult to impossible. It's the equivalent of physician education: those who need it the most shun it. Statistics are dismal and depressing for physicians who care about their patients. The remedy is beyond the scope of this work—maybe beyond the scope of any work.

The logic, however, is unassailable for patients and suggests conclusions most people would denounce: Is it possible that patients:

- Don't care whether they're healthy or sick, or
- Don't care if the live or die, or
- Don't believe that medicine helps, or
- Believe medicine helps, but it's not worth the effort, or
- Exhibit denial, fear, anger, anxiety, loss of face and/or distrust of medical professionals, or
- Suffer from dementia or other mental illness, or
- Can't decide which doctor, relative, or friend to listen to, or
- Think the cost is too high, or
- Can't tolerate the side effects, or any combination of the above.

## Conversations with Patients
## What it's like on the other end of the stethoscope!

### Jacob versus a challenging patient

Jacob Weizman, the octogenarian physician in my novel, *No Cure for Murder*, is an experienced practitioner with great people skills and classical Viennese charm. Although at times abrupt and demanding, he cares for his patients as a loving grandfather. The patients in his practice return the affection. Even Jacob, however, can have trouble with a few patients:

"Who's next?" Jacob asked, as he returned to his office from lunch.

Margaret, his office manager, stared at Jacob, guided him into his office, and sat with him on the sofa.

"With this prolonged prelude," Jacob says, "this next patient must a doozy."

"Amanda Koch has been a patient in at least ten East Bay practices, and for one reason or another they discharged her or she left on her own volition."

"Oh, I can't wait."

Margaret smiled. "It gets worse. She's sued several of our top docs and has submitted complaints against others to the Medical Board of California, or did both."

"I'm waiting for the punch line. There must be a reason why you're willing to subject us to this troubled woman. After all, we're supposed to be friends, right?"

"Ross Cohen, your favorite psychiatrist, thought that you might be the one to deal with her; that's a great compliment."

"Compliment," Jacob laughed. "That reminds me of the Phyllis Diller joke: You know you're old when someone compliments you on your alligator shoes, and you're barefoot."

Margaret laughed. "Still can't take a compliment."

"Ross can keep his compliments. I'll settle for peace and harmony. I've earned it after nearly sixty years practicing medicine." Jacob paused. "Okay. Do we have her medical records?"

"No. She doesn't want you biased against her even before you meet."

"Now, I really can't wait."

Margaret stood, left the room, and returned with Amanda. She was in her early forties with a stocky build and a bulldog demeanor. She had aggressive, spiky, and prematurely graying hair.

Jacob stood to greet her and offered his hand. "Jacob Weizman. It's a pleasure to meet you."

Amanda ignored Jacob's hand and plunked herself into the chair before his desk. "That's a bullshit way of starting this interview."

Jacob smiled. "Who's interviewing whom?"

"If I know anything about this medical community, you're welcoming me like the plague."

"I hate to burst your bubble, Ms. Koch, but until Margaret introduced us, I'd never heard your name."

"Call me Amanda." She paused. "And how did you know it wasn't Mrs. Koch?"

Jacob grinned. "A wild guess."

Amanda barely contained a small smile. "You're wondering why I didn't bring my records?"

"I assume that you didn't want me to see them—at least for now."

"I don't want the crap in those records to bias you, Dr. Weizman."

"You enjoy using salty language, Amanda?"

"I enjoy unambiguous language, Doctor. Does that offend you?"

"Absolutely not. It's better to know what's on a patient's mind than to guess." He paused. "I do need to know our objectives today so I can determine how to proceed. If you're auditioning me to provide medical care, then within my time limit today, let's get to it. If you've already decided to join this practice, then we need to get started with your history and a physical examination."

"What if I'm not ready to decide?"

"That's fine by me. I'll get paid for my time either way."

"That's all you guys ever think about."

"You don't know me well enough to say that. I could have retired many years ago, but I love practicing medicine and still have much to offer to my patients. Can I ask you a question or two?"

Amanda straightened up in her chair and tugged on her skirt. "Shoot."

"Are you happy with your relationships with physicians, and if not, how would you fix it?"

"That's a bit disingenuous, Doctor. You know my interactions with physicians have been disastrous."

"I don't care about the past, Amanda, as long as you don't paint me with the same brush. I don't care who was right or wrong, or who did what to whom. I'm not interested."

"Okay, but this sounds too good to be true."

"I've been around for a while, Amanda. I've seen just about everything one can see in medical practice. I promise to do the best I can and I'll always be honest with you. Do I enjoy practicing with the threat of malpractice litigation or a report to the medical board hanging over my head? Of course not, but you too will find that I have my own demands—reasonable ones, I assure you. We'll deal with them at the appropriate time, and you'll go along with them or move on to the next physician on your list."

"I have my own demands as well, Doctor… or can I call you Jacob?"

"Maybe when you get to know me better," he smiled. "Now, unless I'm mistaken, we'll continue our jousting, and we'll get to business on your next visit, if you choose to return."

"Okay, Doctor. Read 'em and weep. First, I'm no dummy, and if you treat me like one, we're going to have problems. I'm demanding and I want to know everything about my care. I'm a whiz on the Internet, and I'll know more about certain things than you do. If that threatens you, you'll just have to get over it."

"Anything else?"

"Yes. If you or someone in your office hands me a Patient's Bill of Rights, I'm gonna puke."

"Feels good, doesn't it, Amanda?"

"Why, yes it does, Doctor."

They bantered a while. "That's it for today," Jacob said. "I'll get you scheduled for the next available slot. I will have your medical records by then or you'll bring them with you." Jacob stared at Amanda. "It's been a plea…"

"A pleasure, Doctor?"

"It's been interesting meeting you, Amanda."

"Don't disappoint me, Doctor."

"Don't disappoint me, either, Amanda."

# QUESTIONS FOR PHYSICIANS AND PATIENTS

In regards to health, we expect physicians to answer our health-related questions. Patient answers to physician questions are to one extent or another optional due to issues of privacy. As you'll see from the physician questions below, privacy and the omission of essential medical facts may come at a price.

## Tough questions for your Physician

If you're comfortable with your physician, asking questions and stating your concerns will be easier. Doctors and patients need to get along. Both share that responsibility and should use the same skills they employ in developing a successful relationship with friends, family, and colleagues.

**If your physician is not open and available for reasonable questions, find another physician.**

## Samples questions/comments (for reference only).

No patient will ask the majority of these questions, nor should they. Physicians will often feel as if they're undergoing an interrogation if asked too many. Some questions are innocent and reflect a patient's needs. Others may come across as hostile, so don't ask them unless you are comfortable doing so, and you have reason to believe that your physician won't be offended. Nevertheless, keep them in mind and choose the ones appropriate to your situation and your concerns.

1. I didn't understand what you just told me. Please try again.
2. What's my diagnosis? What caused it?
3. How sure are you of my diagnosis?
4. Is this treatment or drug necessary?
5. How does the treatment work?
6. How will I know that the medication or treatment is working?
7. What are the risks and side effects of these medications?
8. Are generic medications okay?
9. What about medication purchased from other countries?
10. What about alternative medical treatments?
11. Are there treatments that don't involve medication?
12. How much will the treatment cost? Will my insurance pay?
13. What's my prognosis? Should I go to work on my bucket list?
14. Is it too late to start ballet or piano lessons?
15. How long will it be before I feel better?
16. If this treatment doesn't work, or I can't tolerate it, are there others?
17. Are you treating one problem or multiple problems?
18. What's the best time to catch you if I have questions?

19. What can happen to me if I refuse treatment?

20. What symptoms or signs should I watch for? Which ones require me to seek immediate care?

21. Should I see a specialist?

22, Are there clinical trials for my problem?

23. How do you justify so many tests?

24. (for women) Can I still have children? Can the medicine affect the baby?

25. Do you have a financial interest in medical, laboratory or diagnostic facilities?

26. How many operations of this type have you done?

## ESSENTIAL QUESTIONS TO BE ASKED OF PATIENTS
### (Questions that physicians should ask, but often don't)

These are serious, but sensitive questions and the physician should prepare the patient for their frankness. The physician needs to tell the patient that the practice asks these questions of everyone, including the clergy and little old ladies. The patient has the right to refuse to answer any and all. The Frustrated Physicians of America (FPA) has recommended polygraphs or lie detectors, but I do not advise them.

• Did you understand what I said? Can you paraphrase it?

• Do you want another opinion?

• Should I explain this to your wife, mother, father, friend, etc.?

• Do you want written information or references (links)?

• Do you use street drugs? What kind? How much? How often?

• Do you use (overuse) prescription drugs? What kind? How much? How often?

• How much do you drink? How much? How often?

• Have you suffered complications from drinking to excess? Blackouts? Tremors?

• Have you been or are you now the subject of sexual/spousal abuse?

• Are you having any problems with your sex life?

• What is your sexual orientation? What specific behaviors? (esp. risky ones)?

• Have you ever sued a physician for malpractice?

• Have you had or are you having suicidal thoughts?

• Have you had thoughts of harming anyone else?

- Do you have trouble remembering things?

- Do you regularly examine your breasts/testicles?

- If you have guns in your home, are they properly secured?

- Do you have an advanced directive for medical care?

- Do you have a health directive? It's appropriate at all ages beyond childhood as everyone is one accident or one severe illness away from needing one if you want your wishes fulfilled.

# MEDICAL MALPRACTICE

While medical malpractice is not an intrinsically humorous subject, a little joke can't hurt. Physicians especially enjoy this one:

A physician was browsing in an antique store when he came upon a statue of a rat. He asked the price and the owner said, "The statue of the rat is $100; the legend behind the statue is another $100."

The man agreed to buy only the statue itself, although the owner warned as he left, "You'll be back for the legend!"

The man tossed the statue into the back seat of his car and started to drive away.

Several rats in a nearby alley began to chase the car. As he went through town, many more rats began to chase the car, until literally hundreds of rats were swarming the car.

Frightened, the man sped toward the edge of town to a bridge over the river. He tossed the statue from the bridge and into the water below. All the rats jumped in after the statue and drowned.

The man, now visibly shaken, returned to the antique store. The owner, seeing him approach, said, "Now, do you want the legend behind the statue of the rat?"

"No," the man replied, "... but do you have any malpractice attorney statues?"

## The unvarnished truths about malpractice suits

- Most patients injured due to their doctor's negligence never file a lawsuit.
- The risk of a malpractice lawsuit has little to do with the number of mistakes a physician makes.
- A bad outcome doesn't indicate malpractice.
- The best doctors are the ones sued more often.
- Many of the worst doctors have never been sued.
- Contrary to the urban legend of doctors protecting each other, the opposite is true. Doctors are responsible for 69 percent of malpractice lawsuits by advising the patients of other physicians to consult an attorney.
- Thirty-eight percent of plaintiffs in malpractice cases are in the health profession.
- Juries decide for the plaintiff in less that ten percent of malpractice claims.

Malcolm Gladwell, in his book, *Blink* explains: Patients file lawsuits because shoddy medical care has harmed them—**AND** something else happened to them: They felt rushed, ignored, or poorly treated.

**The Physicians' Guide for encouraging a malpractice claim.**
**Sue me, please!**

- Provide substandard care.

- Spend as little time as possible with your patients.

- Ignore or dismiss patients' observations.

- Discourage patient participation in his/her own care.

- Don't tell patients your plan for their care.

- Blame greedy patients and greedier attorneys for malpractice claims.

- Blame others, especially patients themselves, for bad outcomes.

- Refuse to explain medical mishaps.

- Refuse to acknowledge actual losses, pain, suffering, and care needed in the future.

- If a physician really wants to screw things up, he'll ask for the judgment of his/her peers since over 70 percent of those reviewing a malpractice claim are critical of the care provided by another physician.

"THE DOCTOR WAS SO GOOD THAT I DIDN'T KNOW THAT IT WAS MALPRACTICE."

## MATCHING PATIENT AND PHYSICIAN
### (Love, hate, or indifference at first sight)

**First Impressions**: Physician-patient relationships are more similar to
how normal people get along than they are different. The charismatic
Marcus Welby and Dr. Meredith Grey of Grey's Anatomy have **it**,
whatever **it**, is. Patients love them at first sight, and often that initial
infatuation outlasts reality and the trials and tribulations of medical
care. Even when reality challenges belief, we still hear things like: Oh
please! Marcus would never do that. Or, Meredith, she's the best, I
never trusted anyone more. Even worse is; oh, you operated on the
wrong kidney; no problem, Dr. Welby, I have another one anyway.
Social scientists call this behavior cognitive dissonance, an
explanation for why people fail to reevaluate first impressions despite
evidence to the contrary.

Medicine hasn't quite gotten to a compatibility analysis equivalent to
*eHarmony.com* yet, but we're coming to understand the principles
that encourage good will and discourage discord.

Specialists in human relations have long believed that people make critical
first impressions within two minutes, while others assert that it only
takes thirty seconds. According to Malcolm Gladwell, in *Blink: The
Power of Thinking Without Thinking,* the decisions may occur much
faster, virtually instantaneously or in two seconds.

Most people swear by their first impressions and rue ignoring them.

First impressions are important—make the best of them.

A young doctor was just setting up his first office when his secretary told him there was a man to see him. The doctor wanted to make a good first impression by having the man think he was successful and busy. He told his secretary to show the man in. At that moment, the doctor picked up the telephone and pretended to be having a conversation with a patient. The man waited until the "conversation" was over. Then, the doctor put the telephone down and asked, "Can I help you?" To which the man replied, "No, I'm just here to connect your telephone."

**Beyond First Impressions:**

**General Considerations:**

An entire literature is devoted to the personality characteristics of physicians and patients and how well the different personalities work together. Like any generalization, it rarely applies to any specific pairing of patient and physician.

The patient's choice of a physician is much like matchmaking, but before getting into details, let me cite the **minimum** standards for choosing a physician:

- He/she is competent.
- Had good training at a reputable program.
- Is on your insurance company's list of providers.
- Has the experience you need in a physician.
- Is the right age, sex, race, and ethnic background (no discrimination intended for patients are entitled to their choices, rational or not).
- Is reasonably close to your home.

Beyond the bare minimum, studies show that patients want their doctors to be:

- Confident
- Empathetic
- Humane
- Personal
- Forthright
- Respectful
- Thorough

Of course, you want to choose the best physician, but that choice is only step one. Developing a working relationship is equally or more important.

# Physician Types

**Type 1: Paternalistic, experienced, a sage**: i.e. Marcus Welby.

Pros: Very comforting to patients. High trust and confidence are positive factors for wellness and improved response to treatment.

Cons: May not be best for patients who want to make their own decisions and/or rebel against paternalism.

**Type 2: Authoritarian, dictatorial.** Have strong bias toward their own beliefs. Tolerates little patient participation: i.e. Dr. Gregory House.

Pros: May have legitimate expertise to a patient's benefit. Putting up with this physician may be "worth it".

Cons: The belief in their talents may be overblown. Putting up with this physician may not be "worth it."

**Type 3. A Partner in Crime, colleague.**

Pros: Empowers patients. Will consider alternative treatments.

Cons: Leaves too many decisions to patient. Deprives patient the benefit of a physician's wider knowledge and experience.

**Type 4. Counselor**.

Pros: Will work with independent patients willing to make their own decisions.

Cons: Medical literature suggests patients using a counselor-type physician do worse with more medical problems and complications. (see below)

## Type 5. Innovator.

Pros:  Willing to try the newest therapy or drug.

Cons: Willing to try the newest therapy or drug. May become too
enamored with new treatments to be objective.

## Patients Types

Before people become patients, they're human, appealing or unappealing, kind or mean spirited, and accepting or rejecting. While the medical literature has tried to categorize patients, it may be better to focus on characteristics that earn some the title of "difficult patients." In an *Archives of Internal Medicine* article in 1999, authors found that physicians classified up to 15 percent of patient visits as "difficult." These patient types include:

- Dependent
- Anxious
- Demanding
- Manipulative
- Self-destructive

Instead, let's focus on patient *behavior* that physicians dislike. Many such behaviors are completely normal unless carried to extremes by patients who:

- Bring in a five-page list of complaints.
- Are rude.
- Don't listen.
- Constantly interrupt.
- Fail to show appreciation for efforts of physician and staff.
- Need constant reassurance.
- Whose symptoms are never relieved by any treatment, or, if, relieved, the patients promptly develop new ones.
- Are self–destructive.
- Who threaten to or employ litigation against physicians.
- Bring meddling and unhelpful companions.

- Lie about their medication or their compliance.

- Have no idea what medications they're taking.

- Who take OTC medications or herbals and don't tell the physician.

- Who stop their medications without telling the physician.

- Reject lifestyle changes important to health such as exercise, smoking, drugs, and demand a pill instead.

- Demand unneeded tests.

- Demand unneeded medications seen in consumer advertisements.

- Omit or delay reporting important symptoms.

- Take medications from prior treatment or from a family member, especially antibiotics.

- Demand medical excuse notes for work, school etc. without proper foundation.

- Demand paperwork, forms etc. without appreciation of physician time constraints.

- Seek drugs unrelated to true need, especially pain medication.

- Who are excessively argumentative.

- Who challenge physicians citing the Internet (Dr. Oz says…)

- Make your own diagnosis and demand a specific treatment.

- Ask another question just as doctor is leaving or say, "by the way, I'm having chest pain."

Phrases physicians hate:

- It hurts all over.

- I always get antibiotics for that.

- I'm sensitive to all medication.

- Medications don't work on me.

- I lost my pain pills (or the dog ate them).

- I don't believe you. Show me the study where…

## BE CAREFUL WHAT YOU WISH FOR

Giving patients exactly what they want, versus what the doctor thinks they
    need is proving to be bad medicine. Researchers at UC Davis studied
    data from a large number of patients and found that the most
    "satisfied" patients:

Spent more on health care and drugs.

Were 12% more likely to require hospitalization.

Accounted for 9 percent more in health care costs.

Were more likely to die.

The reasons for these outcomes are complex, but research does show these
    patients receive more discretionary services, use more drugs (with
    side effects), and undergo more procedures (with their risks).

# THE "MORE IS ALWAY BETTER" PHILOSOPHY

In a world of limited resources, why would we want more done to us,
especially when doing more leads to worse outcomes?

The answers are simple:

- Patients demand more as they equate more with better care.

- Reimbursement systems encourage the physician to do more. Do more;
get paid more.

- The threat of malpractice litigation demands the physician do more for
self-protection.

- Health care management systems are increasingly using patient
satisfaction (or doing more) as an index of physician performance.


Patient satisfaction is becoming the siren song for providing health care
and the Achilles heel for those who embrace competition as the savior
for our costly system. It's perfect; patients get more, doctors get
more, and health management systems glow with competitive
nirvana. Everything's fine until we discover that the costs are
increasing, patients are doing worse, and finally, we're running out of
money—then what?


It's beyond the scope of this booklet to get into more detail on this
complicated issue, except to remind the reader that doing more can
have significant downsides for the patient and the system.

## MEDICAL PROBLEMS THAT PHYSICIANS DISLIKE
### ( Doctors are only human )

While Marcus Welby may feel unqualified love and acceptance for all his patients, real physicians find dealing with certain medical conditions more problematic. If you are a patient with one of these conditions (see below), and entitled, like everyone else, to treatment, it's better to know this up front in order that you and your physician can work together.

Even when patients and physicians act in good faith, certain medical problems frustrate both patient and physician because:

• Treatment is inadequate or incomplete.

• Non-adherence to treatment is high.

• Diagnoses may be uncertain.

• The problems tend to recur.

• They impact on the patient's social skills creating difficulty for physicians (it's difficult to be cheerful and outgoing when you don't feel well). It's too easy to blame the physician.

• A physician's failure to treat or control a disease is frustrating. It's too easy to blame the patient.

These disliked diagnoses include:

- Obesity.

- Alcoholism/substance abuse.

- Anxiety/depression (what we previously called 'neurosis').

- Psychosomatic illness.

- Chronic pain disorders.

- Incompletely understood diagnoses such as fibromyalgia and chronic fatigue syndrome.

- Chronic illnesses, in general.

Effective strategies exist for patients and physicians in dealing with these illnesses, but patients should know up front that it ain't easy. Putting out a contract on such patients is a common suggestion, but it's probably not advisable (although, as a consultant, it may generate more referrals).

## FINDING A PHYSICIAN
## (The right physician)

In the best of worlds, we'd have our choice of physicians. Today, unfortunately, many parts of the country have too few physicians, physician have limited their practices because of volume or their refusal to accept some insurance plans (See Obamacare comments). That doesn't mean that you need to accept any physician willing to open their practices to you. In small towns, with limited numbers of physicians, or in large cities with practices that are full, patients face difficult and uncomfortable choices. How can no care be better than any care? Patients and families must simply do the best they can, but if possible, don't take the easiest way.

### Advice About Finding a Doctor

- Select a physician before you need one.
- BEST: Have a physician you trust refer you to a specific physician/specialist.
- Choose from among friends and associates those most intelligent, critical, and demanding, and solicit their opinions.
- Manage to have a doctor in your family, especially one you love and trust. Get his/her opinion.
- Find a way to meet with a nurse working in a hospital. Nurses know who the best doctors are. Be careful about asking hospitals, medical societies, or physician networks for referrals, as they're likely to send you to practices needing patients. There may be a reason why practices need patients (doesn't apply to new practices).

- Check with the state licensing division regarding complaints against a physician.

- Sit down with a prospective physician. Good first impressions may not guarantee a perfect match, but bad impressions surely do. Trust your gut.

- If the waiting room is filled with unhappy people growing old from waiting, think twice.

- Remember, you're not marrying a physician. If it's not working out, get a divorce.

- On-line rating services may help, but remember human nature; people are more likely to report fault than praise.

# MEDICAL MYTHS

I'm including this section, not only because it's important, but also medical myths are a frequent source of conflict between patients and their physicians.

Few activities generate as much acrimony as challenging established beliefs. To the best of my knowledge and from the review of the literature, these myths cited below need debunking. Truth, however, is an inadequate defense against established belief. Psychologists and psychiatrists call that cognitive dissonance: the mental stress or discomfort experienced by an individual who holds or acts on two or more contradictory beliefs, ideas, or values at the same time. New information that conflicts with these existing beliefs, ideas, or values is especially troublesome.

Here are the myths, the common beliefs, and the information that contradicts them.

I'm girding myself for the torch and pitchfork crowd (patients and physicians).

## MYTH #1: "Overweight" Means "Unhealthy"

One study tracked more than 25,000 men for over 23 years. They recorded who got sick and who died and who didn't. In the end, the study surprised the world by showing that men who were overweight or obese but exercised regularly had half the death rate of normal-weight men who were out of shape. In fact, the study found that being in poor physical condition was far more dangerous than simply being overweight, increasing the risk of premature death as much as having

---

type 2 diabetes, high blood pressure or cholesterol, or smoking cigarettes does

## MYTH #2: Prescription Drugs Are Guaranteed Safe

With intense publicity, few still believe this myth.

About 10 percent of prescription drugs that hit the market are later discovered to cause serious side effects that didn't turn up in clinical trials.

## MYTH #3: Hospitals Are Sterile Houses of Healing

According to the Centers for Disease Control and Prevention, 1.7 million people develop infections while staying in, or immediately following discharge from US hospitals each year. Nearly 100,000 die.

## MYTH #4: Sleep Isn't That Important

It's nearly universally accepted that sleep is important at any age.

## MYTH #5: The Placebo Effect Is Negligible

Thirty-five percent or more of test patients responded as though they had received real treatments. The placebo effect is so powerful that it's the reason we depend on double-blind clinical trials.

## MYTH #6: Too Much Salt Is Bad For You

Based on some very weak studies fraught with uncertainty, salt has been
blamed for a variety of medical conditions—resulting in calls for
extensive reduction or even elimination of it in food products.

This is another misconception unless you are a specific genetically
engineered lab rat. Normal kidneys can always clear salt except in
specific medical conditions related to the kidneys, heart, or liver—for
these, salt restriction is mandatory. In patients with high blood
pressure, some are salt sensitive, others not. A recent study (this
blows my mind) suggested that salt restriction may worsen the
condition in those with congestive heart failure.

## MYTH # 7: Ulcers Are Caused By Stress

Harmful stomach bacteria, rather than acid levels or stress, are in fact to
blame for stomach ulcers. The H. pylori bacteria, believed to be
spread via person-to-person contact, apparently weakens the mucus
lining of the stomach, paving the way for stomach acid to attack our
delicate stomach lining.

## Myth # 8: Old People Sleep Less

It is often heard that the older you get, the less sleep you need. This myth
couldn't be more wrong since it's the complete opposite.

## Myth # 9: Chocolate causes Acne

There have been a lot of scientific studies that prove that there is little to
no chance that chocolate or greasy food can cause acne breakouts.

**Myth # 10: Resting for Back Pain**

Studies have shown that patients that engage in regular activities tend to recover faster and have fewer problems with recurring pain.

**Myth # 11: Over Exertion causes hearth attacks**

Most believe that heart attacks can be caused by excessive exertion, and that rest and a more carefree lifestyle is necessary for recovery. But the surprise is that a less active lifestyle is more likely to cause heart conditions.

**Myth # 12: Vaccines can cause developmental disorders in children.**

This remains a hotly debated issue, despite being debunked in multiple large studies.

**Myth # 13: Catching a Cold in Cold Weather (COULD YOUR MOTHER BE WRONG?)**

People spend much more time indoors in cold weather closer to others. This makes it easier for the virus to spread.

**Myth # 14: You Should Drink 8 Glasses of Water a Day (my wife and her friends are going to kill me for this one)**

This one can be traced back to a 1945 recommendation from the Nutrition Council that a person consume the equivalent of 8 glasses of fluid a day.

Water may transiently make you feel full, but it has no other benefit.

If you're not thirsty, you most likely don't need that glass of water.

## Myth #15: We use only 10 percent of our brains

Advances in medical technology through the twentieth century have
    revealed this to be untrue, as imaging studies like MRI and PET scans
    clearly reveal that no area of the brain is actually dormant.

### Myth # 16: *Medical Diagnosis is always accurate*

When you receive a diagnosis from a doctor, we aren't always 100% sure
    it is correct.

# THE PROBLEMS WITH MEDICAL ADVICE
# (INCLUDING MY OWN)

The most common misperception of all has to do with giving medical advice—after all physicians are in that business. What are the limits of such advice when we know from experience how poorly patients and even loved ones will follow recommendations? When we advise losing weight, getting exercise, stopping smoking, controlling a diabetic's blood glucose, taking medication, how much is enough? And when we advise patients to get the benefits of proven screening procedures such as mammograms, colonoscopies, and regular office visits, how many will comply?

Here are three alternative approaches:

- Nagging: The pain-in-the-ass approach. Persist in giving advice although we know patients will not follow it.
- Surrender: Have your say to the patient and fuggedaboutit—hell, it's their lives, after all.
- Co-opt the advisee. The most difficult approach; urging without nagging, persisting without becoming obnoxious, and encouraging based on a scientific truth; that sincere attempts to change a behavior while failing over and over again, will ultimately succeed, if you both should live long enough.

# INTRODUCTION TO MEDICAL TERMINOLOGY

**What the heck is he/she talking about?**

The Centers for Disease Control (CDC) estimates that 9 out of 10 adults have trouble following their physician's advice largely because they find it incomprehensible. Low health literacy leads to lack of appropriate treatment and poor adherence to recommendations, costing approximately $238 billion a year, and untold pain, suffering, and even death.

The reasons why patients don't understand:

- Use of scientific jargon.
- Confusing instructions from physicians.
- Complicated medical phrases.
- The healthcare provider doesn't have the time, or doesn't take the time to be sure that patients understand.

The move is on at all government levels to simplify language. Note that on October 13, 2010, President Barack Obama signed the Plain Writing Act of 2010 which requires the federal government to write documents, such as tax returns, federal college aid applications, and Veterans Administration forms in simple easy-to-understand language…"

At the present time, 2/3 of Medicaid agencies write health material at a reading level between fourth and sixth grades.

Despite the naysayers, medical terminology is essential for physicians, other health care professionals, and yes, that fact poses a problem for those outside the profession.

When a patient says, "I had a heart attack", the health professional is at a loss to understand. Did that patient have:

A myocardial infarction caused by a blocked artery to the heart muscle, *or*

An arrhythmia, an abnormal heartbeat, *or*

Congestive heart failure, where the heart pump fails to keep up with the body's need for oxygen carrying blood, *or*

Some other heart or lung event?

If the medical record is available, that can help, but often it's not, or it's incomplete and leaves the medical staff confused or worse.

Medical terminology is not a conspiracy against patients, friends, and relatives. There are no physician black helicopters flying in to steal your Internet connection to *WebMD*.

Physicians use medical terminology because it's precise. If one health professional tells another that John Jones had a myocardial infarction, he/she knows exactly what happened.

In any case, patients, families, and others need to understand what's happening to them and to their loved ones. They're entitled to know, and it's the health care professional's responsibility to help them understand to the best of his/her ability. That means explaining medical terminology or using lay words. That may sound simple, but consider:

- Do physicians have enough time and patience?
- Do all patients want such detailed information?
- Will healthcare insurers allow the time needed for such explanations?
- How to explain to those unable or unwilling to understand?

# COMPUTERS AND DOCTOR-PATIENT RELATIONSHIPS

In the United States approximately eighty-three percent of office visits include the use of the computer in the examining room. While physicians, patients, and healthcare systems laud computerization as a godsend to medical care, studies have raised questions about its overall effectiveness at this moment in time.

A 2013 RAND survey of physicians found mixed reactions to electronic health record systems, including widespread dissatisfaction. Many respondents cited poor usability, time-consuming data entry, needless alerts, and poor workflows. Entering and retrieving information into the computer can take a physician inordinate time compared to entering the information in a paper medical record. And, the high number of entry clicks can make physicians feel like data-entry clerks.

A recent *New York Times* article cited the following narrative: A friend of mine, a physician in his late 60s, recently described a visit to his primary care doctor. "I had seen him a few years ago and I liked him," he told me. "But this time was different. A computer had entered the exam room. He asks me a question, and as soon as I begin to answer, his head is down in his laptop. Tap-tap-tap-tap-tap. He looks up at me to ask another question. As soon as I speak, again it's tap-tap-tap-tap." This patient's response—he changed doctors.

Computer errors, changes in workflow, and a huge number of false alarms have physicians longing for the good-ole-days of pencil and paper.

I'd spent a good deal of my professional career in intensive care units where nurses and physicians spent time in direct contact with patients. Now, they spend much time at the computer.

I do not doubt the potential benefits of computerization on patient care, but for the moment, we're in a transition zone, in computer terms— beta testing. Let's enjoy the obvious benefits, but remain diligent to the potential problems.

# SUGGESTIONS

If you feel that the computer's getting more attention than you do, it won't be a surprise that your physician feels the same way. When he or she glances away from the computer screen, smile and ask, "Can I have a moment of your undivided attention?"

# FINDING ANSWERS ONLINE

## Research online, but do so carefully and only at respected web sites

Just because you read something on the Internet, does not mean it's true. If you want to search on specific diseases, diagnoses, and treatments, do not use Google or its equivalent. Such searches will produce a large number of hits, and many, perhaps the majority, will provide inaccurate or even dangerous information. It's better to search reliable sites that contain reputable information reviewed by experts.

**http://www.mayoclinic.com**

**http://www.cdc.gov**

**http://www.fda.gov** (especially good for drug information)

**healthfinder.gov**

**http://www.medlineplus.gov**

**http://www.webmd.com** (user-friendly site)

**http://www.cancer.gov**

Be careful with sites claiming to provide accurate information about hospitals and physicians. Such evaluations are complicated and error-prone.

## CONCLUSIONS
### (Getting along)

In 1936, Dale Carnegie published *How to Win Friends and Influence People*. To date, its sales have topped 15,000,000—not bad for a sales representative for Amour and Company.

To paraphrase his concepts, both patients and physicians should appeal to the other's highest ideals, speak in terms of the other's interests, and allow each other to save face by avoiding unproductive challenges. Common courtesy is the key and you're more likely to enjoy each other's company the next time you meet.

Altruism:

Patients have always taken physician altruism as a given. Sure, physicians have enjoyed status, privilege, and material and financial security, but at the core is the public's belief that their physicians are honest, have integrity, and act on behalf of their patients based on underlying altruism. As the public image and physicians' self-image declines with loss of status, privilege, financial security, and independence, what's left is altruism; hardly a sound basis for a career in our materialistic world. Our best and brightest are proving that, by foregoing the M.D. for an MBA, advanced scientific degree, or heading to Wall Street or the boardroom, or Silicon Valley. In a quote from the prestigious British Medical Journal, "there is a growing feeling that altruism in medicine, if not dying, is at least declining."

Caring about others is not unique to physicians, it belongs to patients as well. Its potential exists in all human beings, but too often, it remains dormant. Altruism may be the one mechanism remaining for patients and their physicians to change the system for the better. If not, the government, acting under the less than altruistic influence of politicians and lobbyists, will make the decisions about medical care for all of us.

# HOW TO SAVE THE RELATIONSHIP WITH YOUR PHYSICIAN
## (If you want to)

**Competent and trustworthy physicians are hard to find.**

If the patient-physician interaction becomes a power struggle, nobody wins. I never thought the day would come when I'd quote Republican Tea Partier, Jim DeMint, but wisdom exists independent of its source. He said: Compromise works well in the world when you have shared goals. I can see no better example than this relationship.

If you know which words will anger or alarm your physician, don't say them.

A pleasant and rewarding office visit today increases the likelihood that they'll continue in the future.

Be as specific as possible when describing your problems. Vagueness not only makes a physician's job more difficult, it turns them off. Don't minimize your problems, especially pain.

If a physician does something extra for you or your family, acknowledge it. If it's obvious that the physician is particularly busy, acknowledge that, too.

Just because you're a big shot somewhere, don't act entitled with your physician.

Leave bad breath or body odor at home (unless they're the problem).

No thoughtful physician expects you to accept everything they say, but unless you have evidence to the contrary, give the physician the benefit of the doubt and keep an open mind.

If you have ten things you <u>must</u> discuss with your physician, start with the most important first.

If you have information about your illness to share with your physician from the Internet, the media, from other patients or physicians, don't present them as a challenge. A simple, "this is what I heard—what do you think," is reasonable.

If you're ethical, expect your physician to be ethical, too. Don't ask for false reports or unjustified excuses.

Complain about the physician's staff with care. After all, he picked them. If they deserve criticism, don't hesitate to voice your concern, but, if possible, bring it first to the office manager or head nurse.

Thoughtful physicians understand that certain people, through no fault of their own, don't get along. Be careful when you complain about previous physicians or consultants for the physician will think, *Am I next?*

Speaking up may be the most positive thing you can do for your health, as the American Society of Internal Medicine estimates that seventy percent of correct diagnoses come from information provided by the patient.

If you think that after a lifetime, you or your physician is going to change, think again. How about making the best of it?

# WHEN SHOULD YOU FIRE YOUR DOCTOR

At first, I thought this section might be superfluous, as it represents the polar opposite of those thoughts incorporated in several preceding sections about patient/physician communication, but there's something about brevity and lists that catch a reader's attention.

Most patients are discomforted by the prospect of firing their physician, and while for most people, it takes dissatisfaction over a prolonged period of time to get to this point, many people do get that far. I have several suggestions:

Make sure that you have engaged the services of another physician first. This is especially important in an environment where the number of physicians is declining or you live in an area where many practices are full and not accepting new patients (i.e. Obamacare).

As many women's magazine have a section entitled, "Can this marriage be saved?" so, too, patients should consider whether or not they could save their relationship with their physician. Too often, the patient and the physician are misreading each other and ascribing unjustified motives to each other. A frank discussion, reality based, may resolve these issues or confirm the patients' suspicion that it's time to cut and run.

## SIGNS SUGGESTING THAT YOU SHOULD FIRE YOUR DOCTOR

- You just don't mesh. You dislike each other.

- You dread coming to the doctor's office.

- He doesn't respect your time or you feel rushed on each visit (you need to respect the doctor's time as well).

- He doesn't explain himself or his recommendations. He prescribes medication without describing the reasons, his expectations, alternatives, and possible side effects. He doesn't interpret lab or other diagnostic tests. He uses too much jargon.

- He doesn't listen to you or value your input. He doesn't show concern for your physical or emotional well-being.

- He doesn't allow you to make the final decisions about your care or pressures you excessively.

- He doesn't seem happy in his work.

- His office staff is unprofessional and/or disorganized.

- Circumstances make you question his competence.

- He acts on his own and doesn't coordinate with other physicians.

- You can't reach him when you're ill or get an appointment in a reasonable period of time. "Doctor's too busy, go to the emergency room" wears thin if it happens too often (many caring practices manage to "squeeze" patients into a busy schedule when needed).

- He's rude and/or condescending.

- He doesn't understand that doing more, even at your insistence, may not help, and might make things worse.

Pay attention to unspoken messages and your own feelings. They are usually significant. It's difficult for a doctor to do his best, or a patient to benefit from care if they are not comfortable with their physician.

# MAKING THE RIGHT DECISION ABOUT EMERGENCY CARE

As long as I'm giving advice, I feel compelled to add this section.

If you collapse and are unconscious, or you've been shot, stabbed, run over by a car, or bleeding to death, you don't need my advice. You must get medical care ASAP.

Physicians know the following urgent situations, but too often they go unrecognized by patients, their families, or friends. People, especially the male of the species, will stretch the limits of denial, perhaps until it's too late to avoid death or severe injury.

If you ask, what can be worse than death, talk to survivors of stroke or severe heart disease. Most believed that it "couldn't happen to them."

**Heart Attack**: If you have crushing chest and left arm pain, break out in a sweat, and you can't breathe, you don't have to be a doctor to know that you'd better head to the ER because it's likely you're having a heart attack. Take note of unusual weakness and sweating even without pain. If you're a woman, you may have instead, "indigestion," jaw or back pain, squeezing discomfort or fullness, or nausea. An early trip to emergency gives physicians the chance to prevent damage from the heart attack or minimize it. Go late, and you may not make it.

**Blood Clot to the Lung(s) (Pulmonary Embolism)**: Sudden shortness of breath, cough, and coughing up blood. Early treatment can save your life.

**Stroke:** Weakness and/or paralysis are the most obvious symptoms. Sudden, and even transient confusion, dizziness, inability to speak, or sudden blindness should raise the specter of stroke or CVA (cerebrovascular accident).

Medical intervention within the first three hours can be life altering to prevent or minimize brain (neurological) damage from a stroke. Sudden extreme headache suggests a subarachnoid bleed. Get to ER immediately.

**Asthma**: Experts say that nobody should die of asthma, but some do. It's so dramatic that everyone but the most obstinate goes to ER.

**Severe Abdominal Pain:** On the pain scale 1-10 (the worst), an 8-10 means get to ER ASAP. Such pain strongly suggests one of several abdominal catastrophes.

**Incarcerated Hernia**: If hernia won't reduce (go back in) with abdominal pain, swelling, nausea and vomiting, it's likely you have a bowel obstruction.

**Blood Infection**: Fever and shaking chill (teeth chattering, not feeling chilly) suggests sepsis, a medical emergency needing prompt attention.

**Spreading Wound Infection**: Sores or wounds suddenly becomes painful and spread rapidly.

**Irregular or Rapid Heart Beat**: Especially associated with weakness, dizziness, or feeling faint, may be life-threatening and needs immediate attention.

Some of these trips will prove to be false alarms, but remember the American proverb: Better safe than sorry.

# GLOSSARY OF MEDICAL TERMINOLOGY

I did not intend that this glossary will be comprehensive. For that you need to go to *Stedman's Medical Dictionary* or something equally complete. I chose these terms because they appear frequently in the lay literature, even when physicians or other health professionals write them. In my own work, I learned early that it's better to have people understand than to be precise.

| | |
|---|---|
| abdomen | belly |
| ablate | to remove or destroy |
| abrasion | a scrape |
| aberration | deviation from normal or usual |
| abscess | a local collection of pus |
| according to (a person or group) | says (a person or group) |
| according to (a study) | based on (a study) |
| accumulation | buildup |
| acne vulgaris | acne |
| acquired immune deficiency syndrome | AIDS |
| acute | sudden or brief |
| acute abdominal pain | stomachache |
| acute rhinitis | runny nose; cold (disease) |
| addictive | habit or dependency forming |
| adipose | fat |
| additional | more |
| administer | give |
| adolescent | teen |
| advantage | plus or pro |
| adverse | harmful or bad |

| | |
|---|---|
| adverse drug reaction | harmful reaction to a drug |
| affect (noun) | feeling |
| aggravate | make worse |
| agitation | restlessness |
| airway | tubes carrying air to lungs |
| alcohol dependence | alcoholism |
| alimentary canal | digestive tract |
| allergen | allergy-causing substance |
| allergic rhinitis | hay fever |
| alleviate | relieve |
| alopecia | hair loss or baldness |
| ALS | Lou Gehrig's Disease |
| alter | change |
| alteration | change occurred |
| alternative | choice |
| amblyopia | loss of sight; no anatomic reason |
| ambulatory | outpatient or able to walk |
| ameliorate | improve |
| amenorrhea | no menstrual periods |
| analgesic | painkiller |
| anaphylaxis | severe allergic reaction |
| anemia | low hemoglobin or red blood cells |
| aneurysm | dilated or weakened vessel wall |
| angina | chest pain from heart |
| angioplasty | balloon repair of narrowed vessel |
| anomaly | defect |
| anorexia | loss of appetite |
| anorexia nervosa | eating disorder with fear of getting fat |
| anosmia | loss of smell |
| anoxia | lack of oxygen |
| anterior | front |
| anticoagulant | blood thinner |
| anti-inflammatory | reduces swelling and pain |
| antipyretic | drug to lower fever |
| aorta | large artery carrying blood from heart |
| aphthous ulcer | canker sore |

| | |
|---|---|
| apnea | no breathing |
| appointment | doctor's visit |
| appropriate | proper |
| approximately | about |
| arrhythmia | irregular heartbeat |
| arterial | artery |
| arteriogram | x-ray of artery with opaque dye |
| arteriosclerosis | hardening of the arteries |
| arthralgia | joint pain |
| arthritis | joint swelling with pain and tenderness |
| ascites | fluid in the abdominal cavity |
| ascorbic acid | vitamin C |
| aspiration | inhaling a foreign body into lungs |
| assist | help |
| association | link |
| asthma | lung disorder with wheezing |
| ataxia | walking like a drunk |
| atherosclerosis | hardening of the arteries |
| atopic dermatitis | eczema |
| atrophy | wasting away of body or organ |
| auditory | hearing or ear |
| auditory hallucination | hearing things that aren't there |
| aural | ear |
| auscultate | listen |
| autoimmune | immune response to own tissues |
| autopsy | examination of body after death |
| axilla | armpit |
| bacterial | caused by bacteria |
| beneficial | helpful or good |
| benign | harmless or not cancerous |
| benign prostatic hypertrophy(BPH) | non-cancerous prostate enlargement |
| bereavement | grief |
| biochemical | chemical |
| biopsy | tissue sample for diagnosis |
| bleeding disorder | clotting abnormality |
| bradycardia | low heart rate |

| | |
|---|---|
| bronchitis | infection bronchial tubes |
| bruxism | grinding the teeth |
| bursa | sac around joint for lubrication |
| caloric expenditure | calories burned |
| canker | an ulcerous sore |
| carcinogen | cancer-causing substance |
| carcinoma | cancer |
| cardiac | about the heart |
| carpal tunnel syndrome | nerves in wrist blocked |
| catheterize | place tube in something i.e. bladder |
| celiac disease | gluten intolerance |
| cellulitis | inflammation of tissues |
| cervical | cervix or neck |
| characteristic | trait |
| chemical dependence | addiction |
| chemotherapy | treating cancer with drugs |
| cirrhosis | scarred liver from infection or alcohol |
| clavicle | collarbone |
| clinician | doctor or therapist |
| closed comedo | whitehead |
| cognition | the process of knowing |
| coitus | sexual intercourse |
| combination | mix |
| comedo | acne bump |
| computed tomography | CT scan or imaging test |
| conclusion | finding |
| congenital | inborn or present at birth |
| congenital anomaly | birth defect |
| conjunctivitis | pinkeye |
| consequence | result |
| contagious | catching |
| contraception | birth control |
| contract (a disease) | catch (a disease) |
| contraindicated | not advised |
| contrast medium | dye |
| contusion | bruise |

| | |
|---|---|
| convulsion | seizure or fit |
| COPD | bronchitis or emphysema |
| correlation | link |
| crust | scab |
| cutaneous | skin |
| cyanosis | blue color due to insufficient oxygen |
| debilitating | weakening |
| defibrillation | shocking the heart to restore heartbeat |
| deficiency | lack |
| degeneration | gradual loss or decline |
| delirium | confusion |
| delusion | false belief or opinion |
| dementia | gradual loss of mental abilities |
| demonstrate | show |
| depression | psychiatric despondency |
| dental caries | tooth decay or cavities |
| dentition | teeth |
| dermatitis | rash or skin inflammation |
| dermatological | about the skin |
| dermatologist | skin specialist |
| detect | find |
| determine | find out |
| detrimental | harmful or bad |
| develop (a condition) | get (a condition) |
| diabetes mellitus | diabetes |
| diabetic (noun) | person with diabetes |
| diagnostic procedure | test |
| dietary | diet |
| differential diagnosis | list of possible diagnoses |
| diffuse | widespread |
| digit | finger or toe |
| disadvantage | minus or con |
| dissect | cut apart |
| disseminated | widespread |
| disturbance | problem |
| diverticulitis | inflamed diverticulum in colon |

| | |
|---|---|
| diverticulum | pouch from wall of the colon |
| drug dependence | addiction |
| dysfunction | problem |
| dysmenorrhea | menstrual cramps |
| dyspepsia | indigestion |
| dysphagia | trouble swallowing |
| dyspnea | trouble breathing |
| dysuria | painful urination. |
| echocardiography | heart imaging test |
| eczema | scaly skin inflammation |
| edema | swelling |
| effective | works well |
| effectiveness | how well (a treatment) works |
| efficacious | works well |
| efficacy | how well (a treatment) works |
| electroconvulsive therapy (ECT) | shock therapy |
| embolism | material blocking blood vessels |
| emesis | vomiting |
| empirical evidence | evidence from experience |
| endocrinological | gland or hormone |
| endodontic | root canal |
| endogenous | inside the person |
| endometrium | lining of the uterus |
| enlarge | get bigger |
| enuresis | lack of bladder control |
| environment | setting or outside factors |
| epidermis | outer part of the skin |
| epidemiologist | expert in disease trends |
| epidemiology | study of disease trends |
| epistaxis | bloody nose |
| epilepsy | having seizures or convulsions |
| episode | bout or attack |
| equivalent | equal |
| erectile dysfunction (ED) | impotence |
| eruption (skin) | rash or breakout |
| erythema | redness |

| | |
|---|---|
| establish | set up |
| etiology | cause |
| evaluate | assess |
| exacerbate | make worse |
| examination | exam or checkup |
| examine | study or check |
| excessive | too much |
| excise | cut out |
| exhibit | show |
| exogenous | outside the person |
| experience (a symptom) | have (a symptom) |
| experiment | study |
| experimental | under study |
| external | outer or outside |
| extract (a tooth) | pull (a tooth) |
| exude | ooze |
| facilitate | make easier |
| familial | family |
| fatty acid | fat |
| febrile | feverish |
| feces | bowel movement or stool |
| fibromyalgia | chronic pain around joints |
| flatulence | gas or fart |
| flexibility exercise | stretching |
| flu | influenza |
| fracture | break |
| fructose | fruit sugar |
| fungal | caused by a fungus |
| ganglion(cyst) | cystic tumor on tendon sheath |
| gastric | stomach |
| gastritis | irritation of stomach lining. |
| gastroenterologist | digestive disease specialist |
| gastroesophageal reflux | heartburn |
| gastrointestinal | stomach and/or intestines |
| gerontological | age-related |
| gerontology | science of aging |

| | |
|---|---|
| gestation | Pregnancy |
| glandular | gland |
| gout | arthritis of small joint, esp. the big toe |
| gynecology | women's health |
| gynecomastia | enlarged breasts in a man |
| halitosis | bad breath |
| hayfever | allergy to plants, grasses etc. |
| health care facility | hospital or clinic |
| health maintenance organization | HMO or health plan |
| hearing impairment | hearing loss or deafness |
| hearing-impaired | hard of hearing or deaf |
| heighten | raise |
| hematological | of the blood |
| hemorrhage | heavy bleeding |
| hemorrhoids | enlarge veins around anus |
| hepatic | liver |
| heritable | genetic |
| herpes simplex | cold sore or fever blister |
| herpes zoster | shingles |
| heterogeneous | mixed |
| high-density lipoprotein | HDL or good cholesterol |
| hirsutism | unwanted hair growth |
| homogeneous | same or similar |
| hormonal | hormone |
| hospitalization | hospital stay |
| hospice | a place/program for the terminally ill |
| immunodeficiency virus | HIV |
| hypercholesterolemia | high cholesterol |
| hyperopia | farsightedness |
| hypersensitivity | allergy |
| hypertension | high blood pressure |
| hyperthyroidism | overactive thyroid |
| hyperventilation | breathing too deeply |
| hypoglycemia | low blood sugar |
| hypotension | low blood pressure |
| hypothyroidism | underactive thyroid |

| | |
|---|---|
| idiopathic | of unknown cause |
| iatrogenic | caused by the doctor |
| immunological | immune system |
| immunotherapy | allergy shots |
| implement (verb) | carry out |
| in vitro | in a test tube or lab |
| incidence | number of new cases |
| incontinence | lack of bladder or bowel control |
| indicate | hint or suggest |
| indicated for | approved or advised for |
| indication | sign or use |
| indolent | causing little pain |
| induration | hardening of body tissue |
| infantile (condition) | babyhood or childhood (condition) |
| infectious disease | infection from bacteria, virus etc. |
| infertility | can't get pregnant |
| inflammation | redness, swelling, and pain |
| influence | affect |
| influenza | flu |
| ingest | eat or drink |
| ingestion | intake |
| inhibit | limit or block |
| initiate | start |
| injection | shot |
| inpatient facility | hospital |
| insomnia | trouble sleeping |
| insulin | hormone controlling blood sugar |
| intermittent | on-again, off-again |
| internal | inner or inside |
| intervention | treatment |
| intramuscular | in a muscle |
| intravenous | IV or in a vein |
| investigate | study |
| investigational | under study |
| in situ | in the body |
| in vitro | in the lab |

| | |
|---|---|
| ischemia | insufficient oxygen supply to an organ |
| jaundice | yellow-looking skin |
| juvenile (condition) | childhood (condition) |
| kidney stones | stones in urinary system |
| kyphosis | humpback |
| laboratory | lab |
| laceration | cut |
| lactation | breast-feeding |
| lactose | milk sugar |
| larynx | voice box |
| lesion | sore or wound |
| lethargic | sluggish, tired |
| leukemia | blood cancer producing white cells |
| limb | arm or leg |
| lingual | tongue |
| lipid | fat or fat-like substance |
| localized | around the (body part) |
| location | site |
| lordosis | inward curvature of spine |
| low-density lipoprotein | LDL or bad cholesterol |
| lupus | antibodies against own tissues |
| macule | discolored skin spot |
| magnetic resonance imaging | MRI or imaging test |
| major depressive disorder | depression |
| malaise | feeling ill |
| malignant | cancerous |
| malignant melanoma | cancer of a mole |
| malingering | faking illness |
| malocclusion | overbite or underbite |
| mammary | breast |
| management (of a disease) | control (of a disease) |
| mandible | lower jaw |
| manifestation | sign or symptom |
| maximal | maximum |
| mean (statistical) | average (statistical) |
| medication | drug |

| | |
|---|---|
| medicolegal | medical and legal |
| meningitis | infected membranes around brain |
| menses | menstrual period |
| menopause | periods end. Estrogen deficiency. |
| metastasize | spread |
| migraine | severe recurring headache, one-sided |
| miliaria | prickly heat |
| mitral valve prolapsed | floppy mitral valve |
| mobility | ability to get around |
| moderate (verb) | limit |
| modify | change |
| monitor | track |
| morbidity | disease rate |
| mortality | death rate |
| motility | movement |
| multipara | two or more children |
| multiple | many |
| muscular | muscle |
| musculoskeletal | muscles and bones |
| mutation | genetic defect |
| mycotic | caused by a fungus |
| myocardial infarction | heart attack |
| myopia | nearsightedness |
| nasal | nose |
| nausea | upset stomach |
| neonate | newborn |
| neoplasm | tumor or growth |
| neuralgia | nerve pain |
| neurological | brain and/or nervous system |
| neuron | nerve cell |
| nevus | mole or birthmark |
| nocturnal enuresis | bed-wetting |
| nodule | lump |
| obese | overweight |
| obstruct | block or close |
| occlude | block or close |

| | |
|---|---|
| occlusion | Blockage |
| occupational | job-related |
| ocular | eye |
| olfactory | smell |
| oncological | cancer |
| oncologist | cancer specialist |
| onset | start |
| open comedo | blackhead |
| ophthalmological | eye |
| ophthalmologist | eye specialist |
| optimal | best |
| orally | by mouth |
| organization | group |
| orthodontia | braces |
| osteoporosis | thinning of the bone |
| otalgia | earache |
| otitis externa | outer ear infection |
| otitis media | middle ear infection |
| otorhinolaryngologist | ear-nose-throat specialist |
| outpatient facility | clinic |
| ovum | egg |
| palliate | to relieve without curing |
| palliative | giving relief but not curing |
| pallor | paleness |
| palpate | feel by hand |
| palpitation | feeling rapid or irregular heartbeat |
| pancreatitis | inflammation of pancreas |
| panic attack | nervous disorder: rapid breathing |
| papule | bump (skin) |
| Parkinson's disease | neurologic tremor and rigidity |
| participate | take part |
| parturition | labor and delivery |
| patella | kneecap |
| pathogenesis | how a disease develops |
| pathognomonic | characteristic of a disease |
| patient | person |

| pediatric | childhood or children's |
|---|---|
| pediculosis | lice, crabs |
| penile | penis |
| peptic ulcer | ulcer |
| perforate | make a hole in |
| perform | do |
| periodontist | gum disease specialist |
| periodontitis | gum disease |
| perioral | around the mouth |
| peritoneal cavity | abdominal cavity |
| persist | last |
| persistent | long-lasting |
| perspire | sweat |
| pertussis | whooping cough |
| pervasive | wide-ranging |
| pharmaceutical | drug |
| pharyngeal | about the throat |
| pharyngitis | sore throat |
| pharynx | throat |
| phototherapy | light therapy |
| physician | doctor |
| physiological | bodily |
| pigmentation | color |
| placebo | sugar pill |
| plaque (artery) | fatty deposit |
| plasma | blood |
| plasma glucose | blood sugar |
| podiatric | foot |
| pneumonia | infection in the lung. |
| podiatrist | foot doctor |
| positron emission tomography | PET scan or imaging test |
| posterior | back |
| postoperative | after surgery |
| postprandial | after a meal |
| practitioner | doctor or therapist |
| preadolescent | preteen |

| | |
|---|---|
| preclinical | not yet causing symptoms |
| predisposed (to) | prone (to) |
| predisposition | tendency |
| preferred provider organization | PPO or health plan |
| premalignant | abnormal, but not cancerous |
| preoperative | before surgery |
| present with | have |
| prevalence | total number of cases |
| prevalent | common |
| preventative | preventive |
| primary | main |
| principal | main |
| principal investigator | head researcher |
| probability | odds |
| prognosis | outlook |
| progressive | gets worse with time |
| prone(position) | lying on your stomach |
| prophylaxis | preventive treatment |
| pruritus | itching |
| psoriasis | skin disease with scaling |
| psychological | mental |
| psychomotor | mental and physical |
| psychoneuroimmunology | mind-body link |
| psychopathology | mental illness |
| psychopharmacologist | psychiatrist prescribing meds |
| psychosis | loss of contact with reality |
| psychosocial | mental and social |
| psychotherapy | therapy |
| psychotropic | mind-altering |
| ptosis | drooping, esp. of eyelid |
| pulmonary | lung |
| purpura | bruising |
| purulence | pus |
| purulent | filled with pus |
| pustule | pimple |
| radiation | x-rays |

| | |
|---|---|
| recommendation | tip or advice |
| recur | return |
| recurrence | return |
| recurrent | repeated |
| reduction | loss or decline |
| reduction(fracture) | put back in place |
| refractory | hard-to-treat |
| referral | sending you to another doctor |
| relapse | slip or backslide |
| renal | kidney |
| renal failure | kidneys not working to eliminate waste |
| resistance training | strength training or lifting weights |
| respiration | breathing |
| respondent (in a survey) | person (in a survey) |
| retardation | slowing down |
| retinol | vitamin A |
| rubella | German measles |
| rubeola | measles |
| rupture | burst |
| scale (skin) | flake |
| scapula | shoulder blade |
| scoliosis | lateral curvature of spine |
| seborrheic dermatitis | dandruff or cradle cap |
| secondary to | due to |
| sedentary | inactive |
| seizures | convulsions, fits |
| self-management | self-care |
| senile (condition) | age-related (condition) |
| senile dementia | Alzheimer's/other related dementias |
| senile lentigo | liver spot |
| sinusitis | infected sinuses |
| skeletal | bone |
| skin tag | extra skin flesh, benign |
| sleep apnea | stopping breathing during sleep |
| smoking cessation | quitting smoking |
| sodium chloride | salt |

| | |
|---|---|
| somnambulism | Sleepwalking |
| specimen | sample |
| spontaneous abortion | miscarriage |
| stabilized | holding steady |
| staphylococcal | staph |
| STD | sexually transmitted disease |
| stenosis | narrowing |
| stent | frame to keep vessel open |
| sternum | breastbone |
| strabismus | cross-eye |
| streptococcal | strep |
| stridor | noise breathing from blocked airway |
| stroke | paralysis from blocked vessel or bleed |
| subcutaneous | just under the skin |
| subject (in research) | person or volunteer (in research) |
| sucrose | table sugar |
| sufferer from (a disease) | person with (a disease) |
| suggestion | tip or advice |
| supervision | guidance |
| supine | lying on your back |
| susceptible (to) | prone (to) |
| suture | sew up or close |
| symptomatology | symptoms |
| syncope | fainting |
| synthetic | man-made |
| systemic | whole-body |
| systemic lupus erythematosus | Lupus |
| tactile | Touch |
| tachycardia | rapid heart beat |
| tarsal | ankle |
| tendonitis | inflammation of a tendon |
| terminal | is going to die |
| testicular | testicles |
| testis | testicle |
| therapeutic modality | therapy or treatment |
| thoracic | chest |

| | |
|---|---|
| thrombolytic therapy | clot-dissolving drug |
| tibia | shinbone |
| tinea corporis | ringworm |
| tinea cruris | jock itch |
| tinea pedis | athlete's foot |
| tinnitus | ringing in the ears |
| TMJ | temporomandibular joint |
| tonsillitis | infection of tonsils |
| topical application | applied to the skin |
| toxic | poisonous |
| toxin | poison |
| trachea | windpipe |
| transient ischemic attack (TIA) | ministroke |
| transmission | spread |
| transmit (a disease) | spread (a disease) |
| transplantation | transplant |
| trauma | injury |
| tremor | shaking |
| ulcer | sore |
| ultrasonography | ultrasound or imaging test |
| URI | upper respiratory infection |
| UTI | urinary tract infection |
| urticaria | hives |
| uterus | womb |
| vaccine | to prevent infectious disease |
| variable | factor |
| varicella | chickenpox |
| varicose veins | enlarge veins in lower extremity |
| vascular | blood vessel |
| Vasculitis | inflammation of blood vessel |
| venous | Vein |
| venous thrombosis | clot in vein |
| ventricular fibrillation | chaotic heart beat |
| verruca | wart |
| vertigo | dizziness |
| vesicle | blister |

| | |
|---|---|
| victim of (a disease) | person with (a disease) |
| viral | caused by a virus |
| viscera | internal organs |
| visual hallucination | seeing things that aren't there |
| visual impairment | vision loss or blindness |
| void | urinate |
| vulnerable (to) | prone (to) |
| zoonosis | disease spread from animals to people |

# MEDICAL SPECIALISTS

**Allergist or Immunologist**: diagnosis and treatment of allergic conditions.

**Anesthesiologist**: administers anesthesia and monitors the patient during surgery. Pain control.

**Cardiologist**: diagnose and treat heart disease

**Cardiovascular surgeon**: operates on heart and great blood vessels.

**Colorectal Surgeon**: operates on colon, anus, and rectum.

**Clinical Geneticist**: diagnose and treat genetic disorders.

**Critical Care Specialist**: cares for patients in intensive care units.

**Dermatologist**: treats skin diseases and skin cancers

**Endocrinologist**: disease of endocrine glands, esp. diabetes.

**Forensic Pathologist**: coroners and medical examiners.

**Gastroenterologist**: treats stomach and intestinal disorders

**Geriatrician**: treats disease of age.

**Gynecologist**: treats female reproductive system and genital tract.

**Hematologist**: treats diseases of the blood and blood-forming tissues

**Hepatologist**: diagnose and treat diseases of the liver.

**Hospitalist**: treats patients in the hospital in place of primary care physicians.

**Infectious Disease Specialist**: Diagnoses and treats infectious diseases.

**Internal Medicine Physician:** prevention, diagnosis, and treatment of adult diseases.

**Nephrologist:** treats kidney diseases.

**Neurologist:** diagnoses and treats diseases and disorders of the nervous system.

**Neurosurgeon:** operates on the nervous system.

**Nuclear Medicine Specialist**: uses imaging techniques to diagnose diseases.

**Nurse-Midwifery**: woman's health care during pregnancy, delivery, and the postpartum period.

**Obstetrician**: treats women during pregnancy and childbirth

**Occupational Medicine Physician**: diagnoses and treats work-related disease or injury.

**Oncologist**: diagnoses and treats cancer.

**Ophthalmologist**: treats eye defects, injuries, and diseases.

**Oral and Maxillofacial Surgeon**: surgically treats diseases, injuries, and defects of the hard and soft tissues of the face, mouth, and jaws.

**Orthopedic Surgeon**: surgical treatment of joints, fractures.

**Otolaryngologist**: treats diseases of the ear, nose, and throat, and head and neck.

**Pathologist**: examines body tissues for diagnosis.

**Pediatrician**: treats infants, toddlers, children and teenagers.

**Physiatrist**: Physical medicine and rehabilitation.

**Plastic Surgeon**: restores, reconstructs, corrects or improves the appearance of body structures.

**Podiatrist**: provides medical and surgical treatment of the foot.

**Psychiatrist**: treats patients with mental/emotional disorders.

**Pulmonary Medicine Physician**: diagnoses and treats lung disorders.

**Radiation Oncologist**: diagnoses and treats cancer and other disorders with radiation.

**Diagnostic Radiologist**: diagnoses and medically treats diseases with imaging techniques.

**Rheumatologist**: treats arthritis and autoimmune diseases.

**Urologist**: diagnoses and treats urinary tract and the male reproductive system.